GOUT DIET COOKBOOK

Delicious Low-Purine Recipes with Meal Plans to Lower Uric Acid and Manage Inflammation.

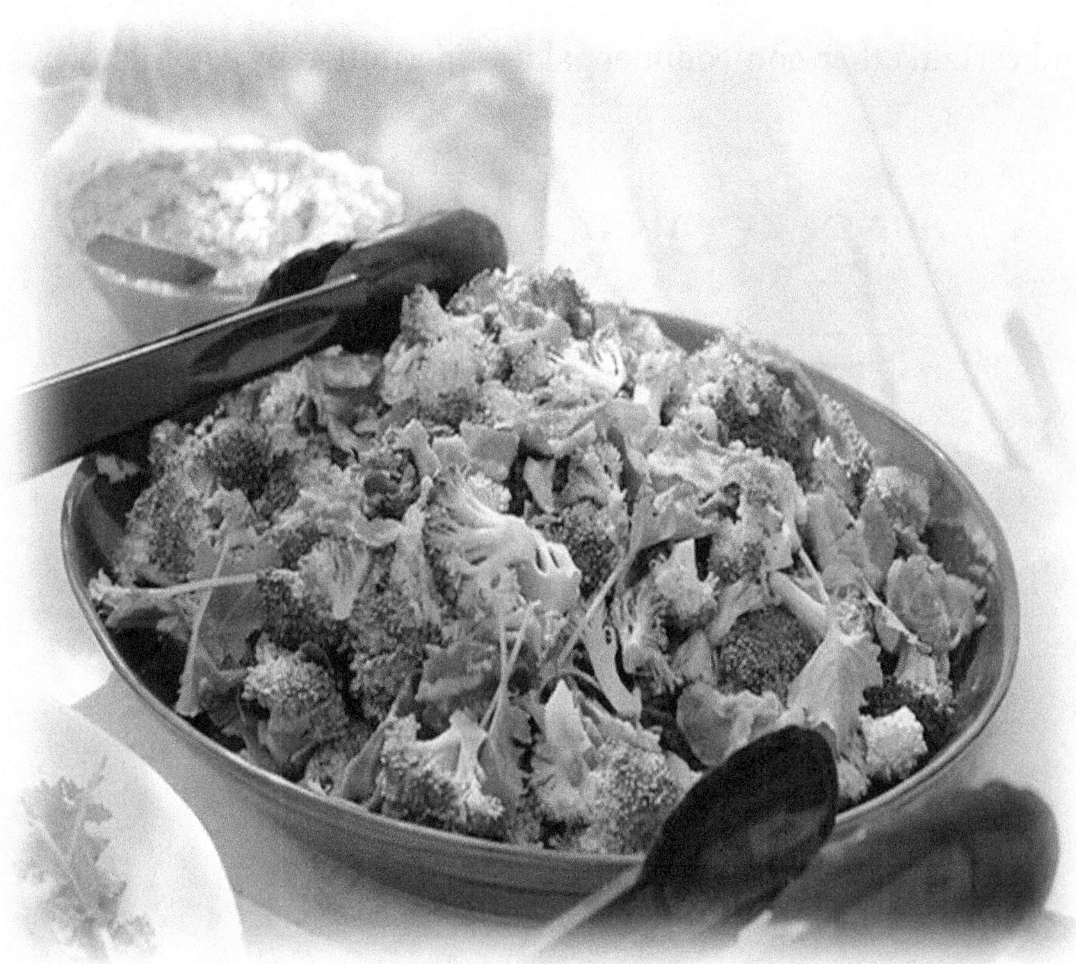

CHRISTIANA WHITE

GAIN ACCESS TO MORE BOOKS

DISCLAIMER

The recipes in this cookbook are provided for informational purposes only and are not intended as medical or professional advice. While the author and publisher have made every effort to ensure the accuracy and effectiveness of the recipes, they are not responsible for any adverse effects r consequences resulting from the use of the suggestions herein.

The information in this cookbook should not replace professional advice. Readers are advised to consult a healthcare provider or a culinary professional before making any significant changes to their diet or cooking practices.

Nutritional information is approximate and should be used as a guide only. Variations may occur due to product availability, food preparation, portion size, and other factors.

The author and publisher disclaim any liability in connection with the use of this information. It is the reader's responsibility to determine the value and quality of any recipe or instructions provided for food preparation and to determine the nutritional adequacy of the food to be consumed.

ABOUT THE AUTHOR

When it comes to tasty and nutritious cookbooks that turn wellness into a delightful journey, Christiana White is the author you turn to. She approaches cooking from a new angle and has a passion for creating wholesome food.

Motivated by her own pursuit of health, Christiana's books on Amazon are brimming with delectable recipes that demonstrate that eating healthily can be both simple and enjoyable. Her creative method makes cooking approachable to all skill levels by fusing entire, simple foods with flavors from around the world.

Readers of Christiana's meals gush about the beneficial effects her foods have on their lives outside of the kitchen. Her books are more than just recipes; they're guides for a happier, better way of life, resulting in everything from more energy to a revitalized passion for cooking.

Come along with Christiana to discover how to turn your meals into satisfying and joyful experiences. Discover the delightful intersection of health and flavor by delving into the colourful world of her cookbooks.

TABLE OF CONTENTS.

INTRODUCTION

Welcome to a world where your kitchen is the front line in the fight against gout. "The Gout Diet Cookbook" is more than just a compilation of dishes; it is a ray of hope for those who have felt the harsh sting of gout's wrath. This book is your ally, guide, and friend as you traverse the treacherous waters of dietary restrictions in search of a haven of delicious, gout-friendly cuisine.

Imagine waking up without the familiar discomfort in your joints, free to move and live without the specter of gout hanging over you. That is the promise this cookbook makes. Within these pages, you will discover the secret to regulating your symptoms with food's therapeutic power. Each composition was precisely designed with one objective in mind: to lower your uric acid levels and prevent gout, all while delighting your taste senses.

From the sun-kissed orchards that produce cherries brimming with flavor and anti-inflammatory properties to the humble fields that provide the diverse and hearty grains that serve as the cornerstone of a balanced diet, we've scoured the earth for items that adhere to the gout diet's strict rules. We've turned these gems into culinary marvels that you can make in your own home.

"The Gout Diet Cookbook" is more than simply a meal plan; it's a lifestyle transformation that puts you in control of your health. We'll go on this trip together, with each chapter serving as a stepping stone to a more gout-free life. So, turn the page and let's start our adventure—one delicious, gout-friendly recipe at a time.

Your journey to a gout-free lifestyle begins here. Are you prepared to take the first step?

CHAPTER 1: THE SCIENCE OF GOUT

Understanding Uric Acid, Purines, And Their Relationship to Gout.

Gout is a metabolic issue rather than a nutritional one. To fully manage it through eating choices, you must first comprehend the underlying science.

Uric Acid is a waste product present in the blood. It is formed when the body breaks down chemicals known as purines, which are contained in your body's cells and the foods you consume.

Normally, uric acid dissolves in the blood, travels to the kidneys, and is eliminated in urine. However, if the body creates too much uric acid or fails to remove enough of it, it can accumulate and form sharp, needle-like urate crystals in a joint or surrounding tissue, causing pain, inflammation, and swelling.

Purines: Purines are naturally occurring chemicals in the body that are also found in many foods. When purines are digested, they degrade into uric acid. Purine-rich foods include certain meats, shellfish, and vegetables, as well as alcoholic beverages, particularly beer, and drinks sweetened with fruit sugar (fructose).

Gout is a kind of arthritis distinguished by abrupt, intense bouts of pain, redness, and sensitivity in joints. The fundamental cause of gout is elevated uric acid levels in the blood, often known as hyperuricemia. Not everyone with high uric acid levels develops gout, although the risk of developing gout increases while uric acid levels remain excessive.

To regulate uric acid levels and limit the incidence of gout flares, it is recommended that:

- Limit your intake of purine-rich meals.
- Maintain a healthy bodyweight.
- Maintain hydration by drinking plenty of water.
- Limit or avoid alcohol.
- Consider eating low-purine foods such fruits, vegetables, whole grains, nuts, and low-fat dairy products.

Lifestyle and Diet Changes: Making lifestyle and dietary changes can have a substantial impact on uric acid levels and gout treatment. It is crucial to:

- Avoid crash diets and quick weight reduction, as they might raise uric acid levels.
- Exercise regularly and keep a healthy weight to lower your chance of gout attacks.
- Be careful of your food choices, focusing on a balanced diet with less high-purine foods.

Understanding these aspects of uric acid, purines, and their effects on gout is critical for anyone suffering from this ailment. Individuals who manage their food and lifestyle can greatly reduce the frequency and severity of gout attacks, resulting in a higher quality of life.

The Gout Diet Can Help Reduce Flare-Ups and Maintain Healthy Uric Acid Levels.

The gout diet is a deliberate eating plan designed to lessen the frequency of painful flare-ups while maintaining healthy uric acid levels.

Reducing Uric Acid Through Diet: One of the primary goals of the gout diet is to reduce uric acid levels by limiting the consumption of purine-rich foods. Purines are converted into uric acid, therefore restricting foods high in purines can prevent the accumulation of uric acid and the production of crystals in the joints.

Hydration: Drinking enough of fluids, particularly water, helps to eliminate uric acid from the body, minimizing the chance of crystal development in the joints.

Weight Management: Maintaining a healthy weight is critical in gout treatment. Excess body weight can raise uric acid levels and heighten the risk of gout episodes. A well-balanced diet, combined with regular exercise, can help you reach and maintain your ideal weight.

Limiting Your Intake of Alcohol and Sugary Drinks, which can contribute to higher uric acid levels, is an important element of the gout diet.

Benefits of the Gout Diet: Following a gout diet can have various advantages:

- Reduced Gout Attacks: Lowering uric acid levels reduces the frequency and severity of gout attacks.
- Slower growth: Eating a well-balanced gout diet can help decrease the growth of gout-related joint deterioration.
- Overall, Health Improvement: The diet promotes overall health by encouraging the consumption of a diverse range of nutrient-dense foods.

The gout diet is a comprehensive nutritional regimen that, when followed correctly, can greatly minimize the likelihood of gout flare-ups while also promoting healthy uric acid levels.

It's a balanced, healthy diet that not only helps with gout but also promotes general health. As with any dietary adjustment, it is important that you speak with a healthcare practitioner to confirm it is appropriate for your unique health needs.

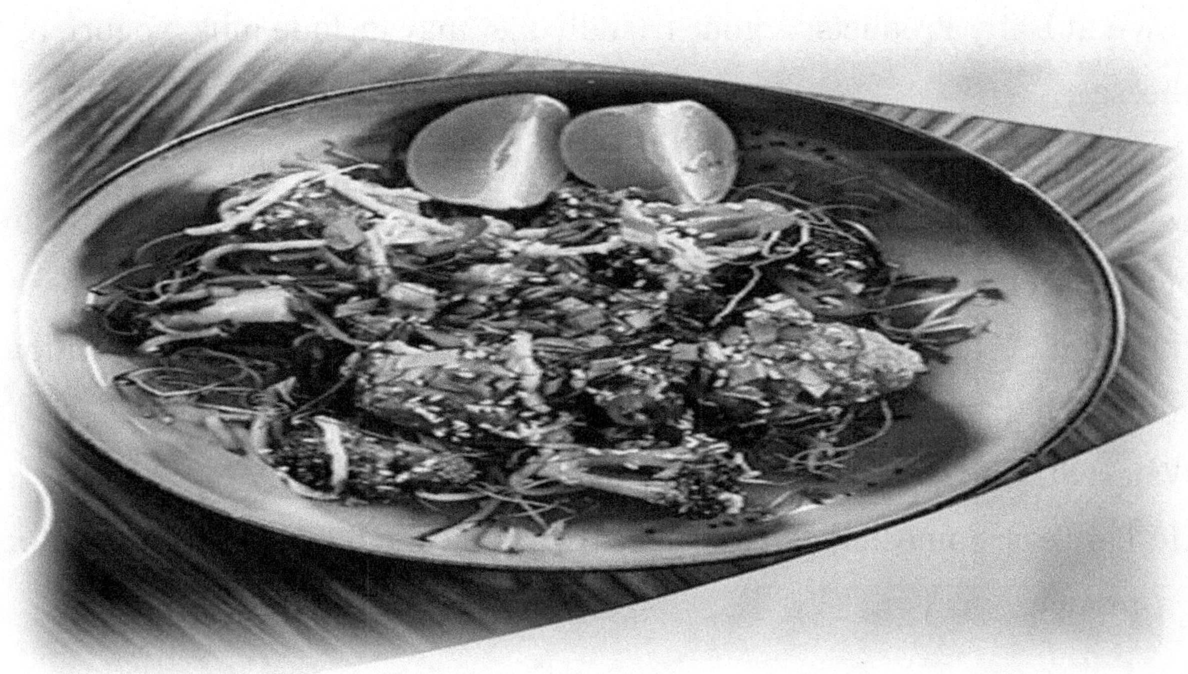

CHAPTER 2: GETTING STARTED WITH THE GOUT DIET

<u>Foods To Enjoy and Avoid.</u>

When managing gout, it's important to watch your diet because some foods can cause flare-ups by raising uric acid levels, while others can assist maintain a healthy balance.

Foods To Enjoy: These foods are often low in purines and are regarded safe for people with gout.

- Fruits and vegetables: Most contain little purines, particularly citrus fruits, which might help lower uric acid levels.
- Whole Grains: Oatmeal, brown rice, and barley are good options.
- Low-Fat Dairy Products: A gout-friendly diet may include milk, yogurt, and cheese.
- Eggs are low in purines and can be consumed in moderation.
- Legumes: Lentils, beans, and tofu are excellent protein sources with low purine levels.
- Nuts and Seeds: When consumed in moderation, these can be a nutritious addition to the diet.
- Water: Staying hydrated is vital for eliminating uric acid.
- Herbal Teas: Some herbal teas can be hydrating and have anti-inflammatory properties.

Foods to Avoid: The following foods are high in purines or can raise uric acid levels and should be reduced or avoided:

- Red meat: Beef, lamb, and pork are high in purines.
- Organ meats: Liver, kidneys, and sweetbreads are especially high in purines.
- Seafoods with a high purine concentration include anchovies, sardines, mussels, scallops, trout, and tuna.
- Alcohol: Beer and liquor can raise uric acid levels, although moderate wine drinking may be less harmful.
- Sugary Drinks and Foods: High-fructose corn syrup and excessive sugar consumption might raise uric acid levels.
- Yeast: Baker's and brewer's yeast contain high levels of purines.

Moderation is key. Some foods containing moderate quantities of purines may not need to be completely avoided, but should be consumed in moderation.

- Poultry: Chicken and turkey have less purines than red meat, but should still be consumed in moderation.
- Vegetables: Asparagus, spinach, and mushrooms are moderately purine-rich but not necessarily restricted.

It's vital to note that people's tolerance for various foods varies. Some gout patients may be able to handle moderate purine meals without developing flare-ups, while others may be more sensitive. Monitoring your body's reactions to various meals and modifying your diet accordingly is critical.

A balanced diet rich in low-purine foods, combined with sufficient hydration and weight management, can help reduce gout flare-ups and maintain healthy uric acid levels.

CHAPTER 3: KITCHEN ESSENTIALS.

Kitchen Equipment Suitable for Those with Gout.

- Nonstick Cookware: This reduces the need for cooking oils, which should be used sparingly.

- Steamer Basket: For steaming veggies, which retains nutrition without introducing purines.

- Blender or food processor: For creating smoothies and soups using gout-friendly fruits and vegetables.

- Measuring cups and spoons: Precision is essential for maintaining optimum portion proportions.

- Airtight Containers: Used to store leftovers and prepared items, making meal planning easier.

- Juicer: For preparing fresh juices from gout-friendly fruits such as cherries and citrus fruits.

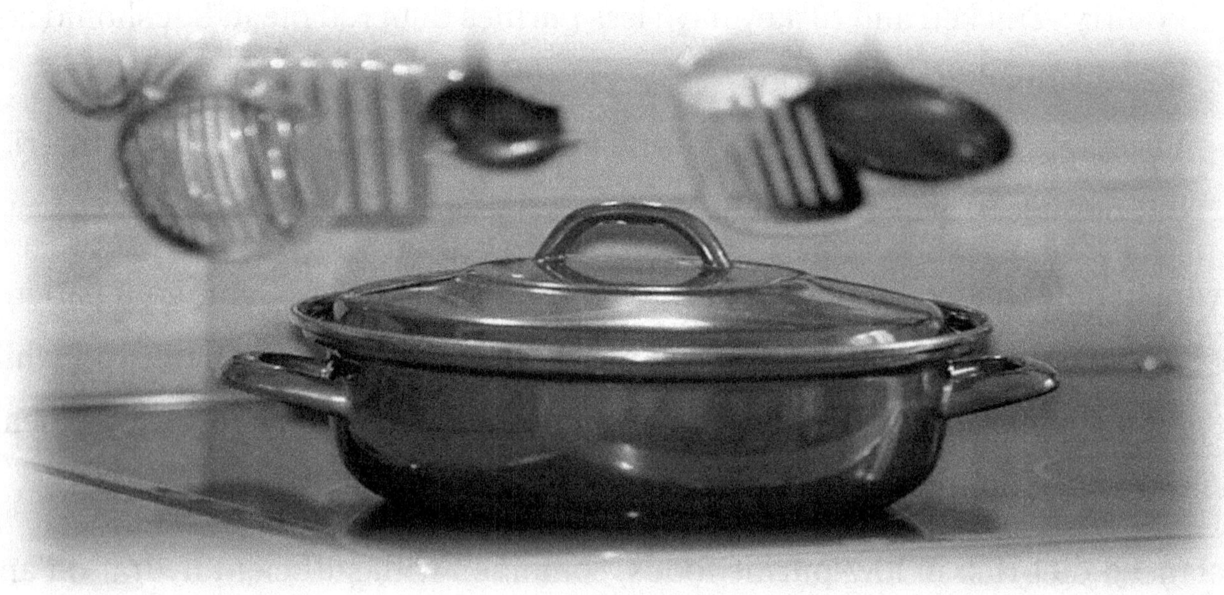

<u>**Shopping lists**</u>

Navigating the grocery shop while treating gout does not have to be difficult. With a little effort and knowledge of smart replacements, you can stock your cart with delicious and nutritious ingredients that promote your health.

Low-Purine Pantry Staples:

- Fruits: cherries (particularly tart cherries), berries, apples, pears, and citrus fruits
- veggies: Most veggies are low in purines and recommended! Concentrate on colorful vegetables such as broccoli, carrots, bell peppers, and leafy greens. Note: Some plants, such as spinach and asparagus, contain significant amounts of purines, but research suggests they do not raise the risk of gout attacks.
- Grains include oats, quinoa, brown rice, whole wheat bread, and pasta.
- Legumes: Lentils and chickpeas can be consumed in moderation. Tofu is an excellent low-purine protein source.
- Dairy options include low-fat or skim milk, yogurt, and cheese (in moderation). According to certain studies, dairy products may help reduce uric acid levels.
- Protein: Eggs, lean fowl (chicken, turkey), and most fish are excellent choices. Limit red meat consumption and avoid organ meats.
- Nuts and seeds: Eat them in moderation (walnuts, almonds, pumpkin seeds).
- Herbs and spices are flavor enhancers that do not include purines! Apply them liberally.
- Healthy fats include olive oil and avocado oil.

Shopping List Tip:

- Plan Ahead: Before you go shopping, make a list to avoid impulse purchases.
- Seasonal Produce: Select fresh, seasonal fruits and vegetables for the best flavor and nutrition.
- Read labels: Choose low-sodium options and avoid processed foods with added sugars or high-fructose corn syrup.
- Shop the Perimeter: Concentrate on the outside aisles, where fresh produce, dairy, and lean proteins are commonly found.
- Frozen Foods: Frozen fruits and vegetables may be just as nutritious as fresh produce and are an excellent way to keep healthy selections on hand.

A gout-friendly diet can be both delicious and satisfying. With a little ingenuity and these helpful hints, you can consume a variety of delectable meals while efficiently controlling your condition.

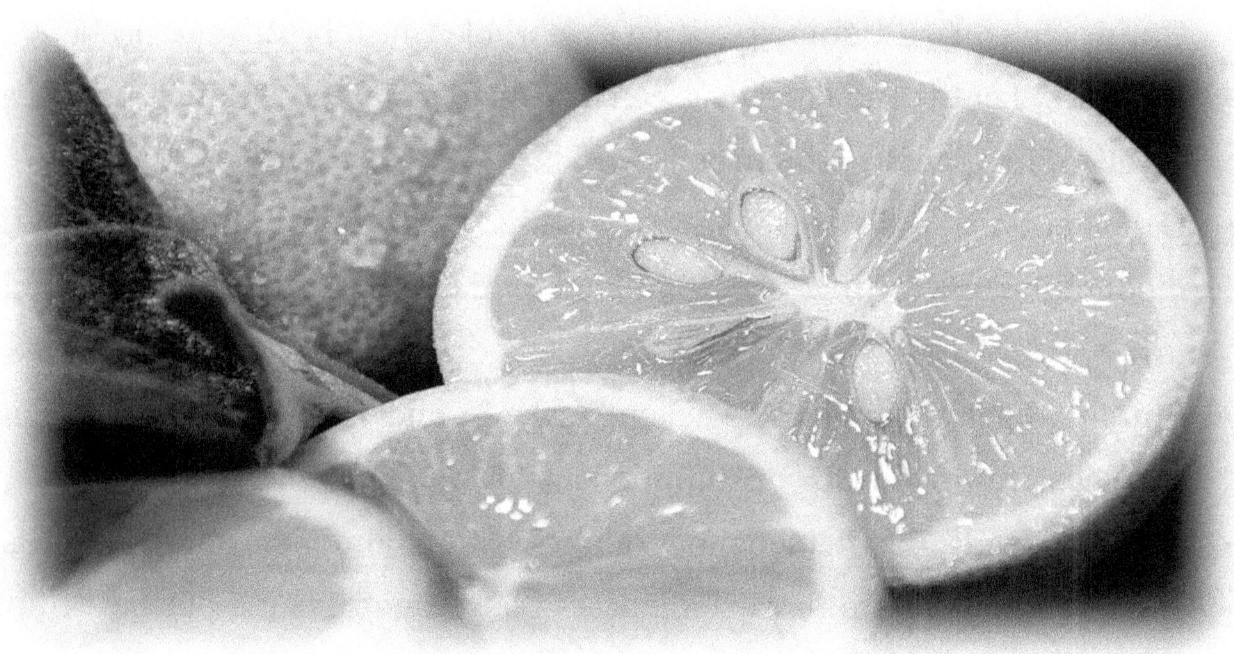

CHAPTER 4: BREAKFAST RECIPES

Oatmeal With Sliced Peaches and Almond Butter

- **Servings: two.**
- **Prep time: 5 minutes.**
- **Cooking Time: 10 minutes.**

Ingredients:

- One cup rolled oats.
- 2 cups water or almond milk.
- One ripe peach, cut
- Two tablespoons of almond butter.
- One teaspoon of honey (optional)
- A pinch of cinnamon.

Instructions:

- In a medium saucepan, heat the water or almond milk to a boil.
- Stir in the rolled oats and a pinch of cinnamon, then decrease heat to a simmer.
- Cook for about 10 minutes, stirring occasionally, until the oats achieve the appropriate consistency.
- Remove from the heat and let the oatmeal sit for 2 minutes to thicken.
- Place the oats in bowls and top with sliced peaches and a dollop of almond butter.
- Drizzle with honey if desired.

Nutritional Information: (per serving) Calories: 295, Fat: 11g, Carbs: 45g, Fiber: 7g, Protein: 9g, Purine Score: Low.

Scrambled Eggs with Spinach and Mushrooms.

- **Servings: two.**
- **Prep time: 5 minutes.**
- **Cook for 5 minutes.**

Ingredients:

- Four big eggs.
- 1 cup of fresh spinach, chopped
- 1/2 cup sliced mushrooms.
- One tablespoon of olive oil.
- Add salt and pepper to taste.

Instructions:

- Heat olive oil in a nonstick skillet over medium heat.
- Cook until the mushrooms begin to brown, about 3 minutes.
- Add the spinach and simmer for 1 minute, or until wilted.
- Beat the eggs in a bowl before pouring them into the skillet.
- Gently scramble the eggs with the spinach and mushrooms until they are cooked through, about 2 minutes.
- Season with salt and pepper to taste, then serve immediately.

Nutrition Information: (per serving) Calories: 200, Fat: 14g, Carbs: 3g, Fiber: 1g, Protein: 14g, Purine Score: Low.

Whole Wheat Toast with Avocado Spread.

- **Servings: two.**
- **Prep time: 5 minutes.**
- **Cook time: two minutes.**

Ingredients:

- Two pieces of whole wheat bread.
- One ripe avocado.
- Lemon Juice
- Add salt and pepper to taste.
- Red pepper flakes (optional).

Instructions:

- Toast the whole wheat bread to your preference.
- Mash the avocado in a bowl with a fork.
- Combine the mashed avocado, lemon juice, salt, and pepper. Mix well.
- Spread the avocado mixture equally over the toasted bread slices.
- Optionally, sprinkle with red pepper flakes for an added kick.

Nutritional Information: (per serving) Calories: 230, Fat: 15g, Carbs: 20g, Fiber: 9g, Protein: 6g, Purine Score: Low.

Cottage Cheese with Pineapple Chunks

- **Servings: two.**
- **Prep time: 5 minutes.**

Ingredients:

- One cup of low-fat cottage cheese
- 1/2 cup pineapple chunks (fresh or canned with juice)

Instructions:

- Divide the cottage cheese into two bowls.
- Top with pineapple pieces.
- For a refreshing breakfast, serve immediately or chill in the refrigerator beforehand.

Nutritional Information: (per serving) Calories: 180, Fat: 2g, Carbs: 16g, Fiber: 1g, Protein: 24g, Purine Score: Low

<u>**Banana and Cherry Smoothie**</u>

- **Servings: two.**
- **Prep time: 5 minutes.**

Ingredients:

- One ripe banana.
- 1 cup pitted cherries (fresh or frozen).
- One cup of almond milk.
- 1/2 cup low-fat Greek yogurt.
- One tablespoon of honey (optional)

Instructions:

- Combine the bananas, cherries, almond milk, and Greek yogurt in a blender.
- Blend on high until smooth.
- If you want a sweeter taste, add honey and blend again.
- Pour into glasses and serve immediately.

Nutritional Information: (per serving) Calories: 165, Fat: 2g, Carbs: 30g, Fiber: 4g, Protein: 8g, Purine Score: Low.

Buckwheat Pancakes With Apple Compote.

- **Servings: two.**
- **Prep time: 15 minutes.**
- **Cook time: 20 minutes.**

Ingredients:

- One cup buckwheat flour.
- One teaspoon of baking powder.
- 1/4 teaspoon of salt.
- One spoonful of honey.
- 1 egg
- One cup of almond milk.
- One tablespoon of olive oil.
- Two apples, peeled and diced
- 1/2 teaspoon of ground cinnamon.
- A pinch of nutmeg.

Instructions:

- In a bowl, combine the buckwheat flour, baking powder, and salt.
- In a separate dish, whisk together the honey, egg, and almond milk.
- Mix together the wet and dry ingredients until a batter forms.
- Heat a nonstick pan over medium heat and brush with olive oil.
- Pour 1/4 cup batter onto each pancake and heat until bubbles appear on the surface, then flip and cook until golden brown.
- For the compote, combine the diced apples, cinnamon, and nutmeg in a saucepan with a splash of water. Simmer until the apples have softened.
- Serve the pancakes topped with warm apple compote.

Nutritional Information: calories: 320, fat: 8g, carbs: 55g, fiber: 8g, protein: 10g, purine score: low

Quinoa Porridge with Almonds and Blueberries.

- **Servings: two.**
- **Prep time: 5 minutes.**
- **Cook time: 15 minutes.**

Ingredients:

- 1/2 cup washed quinoa.
- One cup of water.
- One cup of almond milk.
- One-half cup blueberries
- One-quarter cup chopped almonds
- One spoonful of honey or maple syrup

Instructions:

- In a saucepan, combine the quinoa and water and heat till boiling.
- Reduce the heat to low, cover, and simmer for 15 minutes, or until the quinoa is done.
- Stir in the almond milk and cook until heated through.
- Top the porridge with blueberries, almonds, and a drizzle of honey or maple syrup.

Nutritional Information: calories: 285, fat: 9g, carbs: 44g, fiber: 6g, protein: 8g, purine score: low.

Baked Sweet Potatoes with Cinnamon and Nutmeg.

- **Servings: two.**
- **Prep time: 5 minutes.**
- **Cook for 45 minutes.**

Ingredients:

- Two medium sweet potatoes.
- 1/2 teaspoon of ground cinnamon.
- A pinch of nutmeg.
- One spoonful of honey or maple syrup

Instructions:

- Preheat your oven to 400°F (200°C).
- Pierce the sweet potatoes with a fork and arrange on a baking sheet.
- Bake for 45 minutes, or until tender.
- Cut the sweet potatoes open and sprinkle with cinnamon and nutmeg.
- Drizzle with honey or maple syrup before serving.

Nutritional Information: Calories: 195, fat: 0.3g, carbs: 46g, fiber: 7g, protein: 2g, purine score: low.

<u>Chia Seed Pudding with Fresh Fruit</u>

- **Servings: two.**
- **Prep time is 5 minutes (plus soaking time).**

Ingredients:

- 1/4 cup of chia seeds.
- One cup of almond milk.
- One spoonful of honey or maple syrup
- 1/2 cup mixed fresh fruit (such as berries, kiwi, and banana)

Instructions:

- In a bowl, combine the chia seeds, almond milk, and honey or maple syrup.
- Refrigerate the mixture for at least 2 hours or overnight until it reaches pudding consistency.
- Stir the pudding and adjust the sweetness as needed.
- Serve topped with fresh fruit.

Nutritional Information: Calories: 180, fat: 9g, carbs: 24g, fiber: 10g, protein: 5g, purine score: low.

CHAPTER 5: LUNCH RECIPES.

<u>Mixed Salad with Cottage Cheese and Chives.</u>

- **Servings: two.**
- **Prep time: 10 minutes.**

Ingredients:

- Two cups mixed salad greens.
- 1/2 cup cherry tomatoes, cut in half
- 1/2 cucumber, sliced
- 1/2 cup of low-fat cottage cheese
- 2 tablespoons coarsely chopped chives.
- One tablespoon of olive oil.
- One tablespoon of balsamic vinegar.
- Add salt and pepper to taste.

Instructions:

- In a large bowl, combine the mixed salad greens, cherry tomatoes, and cucumber slices.
- To make the dressing, combine the olive oil and balsamic vinegar in a separate small bowl and season with salt and pepper.
- Pour the dressing over the salad and gently toss to coat.
- Top the salad with a scoop of cottage cheese.
- Garnish with chopped chives.

Nutritional Information: Calories: 150, Fat: 7g, Carbs: 10g, Fiber: 2g, Protein: 12g, Purine Score: Low.

Egg Salad Sandwich on Whole Wheat Bread

- **Servings: two.**
- **Prep time: 10 minutes.**
- **Cooking Time: 10 minutes.**

Ingredients:

- 4 hardboiled eggs, peeled and diced.
- Two tablespoons of low-fat mayonnaise.
- One tablespoon mustard.
- 1/4 cup finely chopped celery.
- Add salt and pepper to taste.
- Four pieces of whole wheat bread.
- Lettuce leaves

Instructions:

- In a bowl, combine the chopped hard-boiled eggs, mayonnaise, mustard, and celery.
- Season with salt and pepper to taste and stir thoroughly.
- Spread lettuce leaves on two slices of whole wheat bread.
- Spread the egg salad mixture over the lettuce.
- Add the remaining slices of bread to make sandwiches.

Nutritional Information: calories: 320, fat: 15g, carbs: 27g, fiber: 5g, protein: 19g, purine score: low.

<u>Lentil Soup with Carrots and Celery</u>

- **Servings: four.**
- **Prep time: 10 minutes.**
- **Cook for 30 minutes.**

Ingredients:

- 1 cup washed lentils.
- Four cups of veggie broth.
- One carrot, chopped
- One stalk of celery, chopped
- 1 onion, diced
- 2 garlic cloves, minced
- One tablespoon of olive oil.
- One teaspoon thyme.
- Add salt and pepper to taste.

Instructions:

- Heat the olive oil in a big pot over medium heat.
- Sauté the onion and garlic until transparent.
- Add the carrots and celery and simmer for a further 5 minutes.
- Add the veggie broth and bring to a boil.
- Add the lentils and thyme, then lower the heat to a simmer.
- Cook for approximately 25 minutes, or until lentils are cooked.
- Add salt and pepper to taste.
- Serve hot.

Nutritional Information: Calories: 240, Fat: 4g, Carbs: 38g, Fiber: 16g, Protein: 14g, Purine Score: Low.

<u>Grilled Chicken Breast and Steamed Vegetables</u>

- **Servings: two.**
- **Prep time: 5 minutes.**
- **Cook time: 20 minutes.**

Ingredients:

- Two boneless, skinless chicken breasts.
- One tablespoon of olive oil.
- Add salt and pepper to taste.
- 1 cup of broccoli florets.
- 1 cup chopped carrots.
- 1 cup sliced zucchini.

Instructions:

- Preheat the grill to medium-high.
- Brush olive oil on the chicken breasts and season with salt and pepper.
- Grill the chicken for 10 minutes on each side, or until thoroughly done.
- While the chicken grills, steam the broccoli, carrots, and zucchini until soft, about 5-7 minutes.
- Serve the grilled chicken beside the steamed vegetables on the side.

Nutritional Information: Calories: 295, Fat: 9g, Carbs: 10g, Fiber: 4g, Protein: 44g, Purine Score: Low.

<u>Quinoa & Black Bean Salad</u>

- **Servings: four.**
- **Prep time: 15 minutes.**
- **Cook time: 20 minutes.**

Ingredients:

- One cup quinoa.
- Two glasses of water.
- One can (15 oz) of black beans, drained and rinsed
- One red bell pepper, chopped
- 1/4 cup fresh cilantro, chopped
- 1/4 cup of lime juice.
- Two teaspoons of olive oil.
- Add salt and pepper to taste.

Instructions:

- Rinse the quinoa in cool water until it runs clean.
- In a saucepan, heat 2 cups of water till boiling. Add the quinoa, reduce the heat to low, cover, and cook for 15-20 minutes, until the water is absorbed.
- Fluff the cooked quinoa with a fork and let it cool.
- In a large bowl, combine the chilled quinoa, black beans, and diced red bell pepper.
- In a small bowl, combine lime juice, olive oil, salt, and pepper to make a dressing.
- Pour the dressing over the quinoa and toss to incorporate.
- Garnish with fresh cilantro before serving.

Nutritional Information: calories: 320, fat: 7g, carbs: 52g, fiber: 10g, protein: 12g, purine score: low

Vegetable Wrap with Hummus and Cucumber

- **Servings: two.**
- **Prep time: 10 minutes.**

Ingredients:

- Two whole wheat tortillas.
- 1/2 cup hummus.
- One cucumber, thinly sliced
- 1 grated carrot.
- 1/2 red bell pepper, thinly sliced
- One handful of mixed greens.

Instructions:

- Arrange the whole wheat tortillas on a level surface.
- Spread a layer of hummus over each tortilla.
- Arrange cucumber slices, shredded carrot, red bell pepper slices, and mixed greens evenly on the tortillas.
- Roll the tortillas tightly, tucking the edges in.
- Cut the wraps in half and serve.

Nutritional Information: Calories: 260, fat: 8g, carbohydrates: 40g, fiber: 8g, protein: 10g, purine score: low

<u>Baked Cod with Lemon and Dill.</u>

- **Servings: two.**
- **Prep time: 5 minutes.**
- **Cook time: 15 minutes.**

Ingredients:

- Two cod fillets, 6 ounces apiece.
- One lemon, cut
- 2 teaspoons fresh dill, chopped.
- One tablespoon of olive oil.
- Add salt and pepper to taste.

Instructions:

- Preheat your oven to 400°F (200°C).
- Arrange the fish fillets on a baking pan lined with parchment paper.
- Drizzle olive oil over the cod and season with salt and pepper.
- Garnish each fillet with lemon slices and fresh dill.
- Bake in a preheated oven for 12-15 minutes, or until the fish easily flaked with a fork.

Nutritional Information: Calories: 190, Fat: 5g, Carbs: 0g, Fiber: 0g, Protein: 31g, Purine Score: Low

<u>Stuffed Bell Peppers with Brown Rice and Vegetables.</u>

- **Servings: four.**
- **Prep time: 20 minutes.**
- **Cook for 30 minutes.**

Ingredients:

- 4 bell peppers with tops cut off and seeds removed
- One cup of cooked brown rice.
- 1 zucchini, diced
- 1/2 cup of corn kernels.
- 1/2 onion, diced
- 1 clove garlic, minced
- One cup of tomato sauce.
- One teaspoon of oregano.
- One tablespoon of olive oil.
- Add salt and pepper to taste.

Instructions:

- Preheat the oven to 350°F/175°C.
- In a skillet, heat the olive oil over medium heat. Sauté the onion and garlic until transparent.
- Cook an additional 5 minutes after adding the zucchini and corn.
- Add the cooked brown rice, tomato sauce, and oregano. Season with salt and pepper.
- Fill each bell pepper with the rice-vegetable mixture.
- Transfer the stuffed peppers to a baking tray and bake for 30 minutes, or until soft.

Nutritional Information: Calories: 250, fat: 4g, carbs: 48g, fiber: 8g, protein: 6g, purine score: low.

CHAPTER 6: DINNER RECIPES.

<u>Grilled Salmon with A Side of Asparagus</u>

- **Servings: two.**
- **Prep time: 10 minutes.**
- **Cook time: 15 minutes.**

Ingredients:

- Two salmon fillets, 6 ounces apiece.
- 1 bunch of asparagus, with ends trimmed
- One tablespoon of olive oil.
- One lemon, cut
- Add salt and pepper to taste.
- Fresh dill as garnish

Instructions:

- Preheat the grill to medium-high.
- Coat the salmon fillets and asparagus with olive oil. Season with salt and pepper.
- Place the salmon on the grill, skin side down, and arrange the asparagus around.
- Grill the salmon for 6-8 minutes per side, or until readily flaked with a fork.
- Grill the asparagus for 5 minutes, turning periodically, until tender and faintly browned.
- Top the grilled salmon and asparagus with lemon slices and fresh dill.

Nutritional Information: calories: 345, fat: 19g, carbs: 6g, fiber: 3g, protein: 35g, purine score: low.

<u>Chicken And Broccoli Casserole with Cherries and Almonds</u>

- **Servings: four.**
- **Prep time: 20 minutes.**
- **Cook for 30 minutes.**

Ingredients:

- 2 cups cooked chicken breast, diced
- Two cups broccoli florets.
- 1/2 cup of dried cherries.
- One-quarter cup chopped almonds
- One cup of low-fat Greek yogurt
- 1/2 cup of low-sodium chicken broth
- One teaspoon of garlic powder.
- Add salt and pepper to taste.

Instructions:

- Preheat your oven to 375°F (190°C).
- In a large bowl, combine the Greek yogurt, chicken broth, garlic powder, salt, and pepper.
- Stir in the cooked chicken, broccoli, dried cherries, and almonds.
- Place the mixture in a greased baking dish.
- Bake for 30 minutes, or until the casserole bubbles and the broccoli is cooked.
- Serve hot.

Nutritional Information: Calories: 280, Fat: 8g, Carbs: 18g, Fiber: 3g, Protein: 34g, Purine Score: Low.

Vegetable Stir-Fry with Tofu

- **Servings: four.**
- **Prep time: 15 minutes.**
- **Cooking Time: 10 minutes.**

Ingredients:

- One block of firm tofu, drained and cubed
- Two cups of mixed vegetables (bell peppers, carrots, snap peas)
- 2 teaspoons of soy sauce (low sodium)
- One tablespoon of sesame oil.
- 1 teaspoon grated ginger.
- 1 clove garlic, minced
- One spoonful of cornstarch.
- One-quarter cup water

Instructions:

- Cook the sesame oil in a large skillet or wok over medium-high heat.
- Stir-fry the tofu cubes until golden brown, about 5 minutes. Remove and set aside.
- In the same skillet, combine the mixed vegetables, ginger, and garlic. Stir-fry for five minutes.
- In a small bowl, combine soy sauce, cornstarch, and water.
- Pour the sauce into the skillet with the vegetables and heat to a simmer.
- Return the tofu to the skillet and combine everything until the sauce thickens.
- Serve hot.

Nutritional Information: Calories: 150, fat: 7g, carbs: 10g, fiber: 3g, protein: 12g, purine score: low.

<u>**Baked Trout with Herbal Seasoning**</u>

- **Servings: two.**
- **Prep time: 5 minutes.**
- **Cook time: 20 minutes.**

Ingredients:

- 2 trout fillets (6 ounces each)
- One tablespoon of olive oil.
- One teaspoon dried thyme.
- One teaspoon of dried rosemary
- Add salt and pepper to taste.
- Lemon wedges to serve.

Instructions:

- Preheat your oven to 375°F (190°C).
- Arrange the fish fillets on a baking pan lined with parchment paper.
- Coat each fillet in olive oil and season with thyme, rosemary, salt, and pepper.
- Bake for 20 minutes, or until the fish flaked easily with a fork.
- Serve with lemon wedges.

Nutritional Information: Calories: 290, Fat: 14g, Carbs: 0g, Fiber: 0g, Protein: 38g, Purine Score: Low

Roasted Turkey Breast and Green Beans

- **Servings: four.**
- **Prep time: 10 minutes.**
- **Cook for 30 minutes.**

Ingredients:

- 2-pound turkey breast
- 1-pound green beans, trimmed
- Two teaspoons of olive oil.
- Add salt and pepper to taste.
- One teaspoon dried thyme.

Instructions:

- Preheat the oven to 350°F/175°C.
- Season turkey breast with salt, pepper, and thyme.
- Put the turkey in a roasting pan and drizzle with 1 tablespoon olive oil.
- Roast in the oven for 25-30 minutes, or until the internal temperature reaches 165°F (74°C).
- While the turkey roasts, blanch the green beans in boiling water for 3-4 minutes before draining.
- Mix the green beans with the remaining olive oil, salt, and pepper.
- Add the green beans to the roasting pan in the last 10 minutes of cooking the turkey.
- Serve the turkey sliced, with green beans on the side.

Nutritional Information: Calories: 345, Fat: 9g, Carbs: 10g, Fiber: 4g, Protein: 55g, Purine Score: Low.

<u>**Shrimp and Vegetable Kabobs**</u>

- **Servings: four.**
- **Prep time: 20 minutes.**
- **Cooking Time: 10 minutes.**

Ingredients:

- 1 pound of big shrimp, peeled and deveined
- One zucchini sliced into bits.
- 1 red bell pepper chopped into bits.
- 1 yellow bell pepper chopped into bits.
- Two teaspoons of olive oil.
- One lemon, juiced
- One teaspoon of garlic powder.
- Add salt and pepper to taste.

Instructions:

- Preheat the grill to medium-high heat.
- In a bowl, combine the olive oil, lemon juice, garlic powder, salt, and pepper.
- Toss the shrimp and vegetables in the marinade until evenly covered.
- Thread the shrimp and vegetables on skewers.
- Grill the kabobs for 2-3 minutes per side, or until the shrimp turn pink and opaque.
- Serve the kabobs fresh from the grill.

Nutritional Information: Calories: 225, fat: 10g, carbs: 8g, fiber: 2g, protein: 26g, purine score: low.

<u>Lentils and Vegetable Curry</u>

- **Servings: four.**
- **Prep time: 15 minutes.**
- **Cook for 30 minutes.**

Ingredients:

- One cup red lentil.
- One large carrot, chopped
- One large potato, diced
- 1 onion, chopped
- 2 garlic cloves, minced
- One tablespoon of curry powder.
- One teaspoon of ground cumin
- Four cups of veggie broth.
- One can (14 ounces) of diced tomatoes
- One cup spinach leaf.
- Salt to taste.

Instructions:

- Rinse the lentils thoroughly in cold water until they run clear.
- In a large pot, cook the onion and garlic until transparent.
- Stir in the curry powder and cumin for approximately a minute, until aromatic.
- Combine the lentils, carrot, potato, vegetable broth, and diced tomatoes in the pot.

- Bring to a boil, then lower the heat and simmer for 20 minutes, or until the lentils and veggies are cooked.
- Add the spinach and simmer until wilted.
- Season with salt to taste, and serve warm.

Nutritional Information: Calories: 260, fat: 2g, carbohydrates: 48g, fiber: 14g, protein: 14g, purine score: low

CHAPTER 7: SNACKS AND SIDES.

<u>Carrot And Celery Sticks with Almond Butter.</u>

- **Servings: two.**
- **Prep time: 5 minutes.**

Ingredients:

- 2 large carrots peeled and sliced into sticks.
- Cut 2 large celery stalks into sticks.
- One-quarter cup almond butter

Instructions:

- Arrange the carrot and celery sticks on a platter.
- Serve alongside almond butter for dipping.

Nutritional Information: Calories: 164, Fat: 12g, Carbs: 12g, Fiber: 3g, Protein: 5g, Purine Score: Low

Cherry Walnut Smoothie

- **Serves: 1**
- **Prep time: 5 minutes.**

Ingredients:

- 1 cup ripe, pitted cherries
- 3/4 cup unsweetened almond milk.
- 2 tablespoons of raw walnuts, chopped
- One ripe banana, peeled and frozen

Instructions:

- Combine all ingredients in a blender.
- Blend until smooth and creamy.
- Serve immediately.

Nutritional Information: Calories: 307, Fat: 12g, Carbs: 48g, Protein: 6g, Fiber: 8g, Sugar: 32g, Purine Score: Low.

<u>**Greek Yogurt with Honey and Walnuts.**</u>

- **Serves: 1**
- **Prep time: 2 minutes.**

Ingredients:

- 150 grams of full-fat Greek yogurt.
- Two teaspoons of honey.
- Chopped walnuts.

Instructions:

- In a mixing bowl, combine the yogurt and whisk until smooth.
- Garnish with honey and chopped walnuts.
- Serve immediately.

Nutritional Information: calories: 372, fat: 18g, carbs: 9.8g, purine score: low.

<u>Fresh Fruit Salad.</u>

- **Servings: six.**
- **Prep time: 10 minutes.**

Ingredients:

- One pint of fresh raspberries.
- One pint of fresh strawberries, quartered
- One pint of fresh blueberries.
- 2 cups of grapes, halved
- 2 cups fresh pineapple chunks.
- Fresh mint leaves (optional).
- One orange (for juice and zest).

Instructions:

- Place all of the fruit in a big bowl.
- If desired, garnish with chopped fresh mint leaves.
- Zest some orange over the bowl, then squeeze some fresh orange juice on top.
- Serve immediately or chill till later.

Nutritional Information: Calories: 183, Fat: 0g, Carbs: 47g, Fiber: 8g, Protein: 2g, Purine Score: Low

<u>Almonds And Sunflower Seeds.</u>

- **Serves: 12**
- **Prep time: 5 minutes.**

Ingredients:

- Three parts raw linseed (flaxseed).
- Two parts raw sunflower seeds.
- One-part raw almonds.

Instructions:

- Combine linseed, sunflower seeds, and almonds in a blender or food processor.
- Blend on high speed for 10-20 seconds, or until finely ground.
- Refrigerate in a sealed jar.

Nutritional Information: Calories: 43 (per tablespoon); Fat: 3g; Carbs: 2g; Fiber: 1g; Protein: 1.5g; Purine Score: Low.

<u>Baked Kale Chips</u>

- **Servings: six.**
- **Prep time: 10 minutes.**
- **Cook time: 20 minutes.**

Ingredients:

- 1 ½ cups washed, dried kale with rough stems removed and shredded.
- 1 teaspoon of olive oil.
- Fine salt, to taste.

Instructions:

- Preheat your oven to 140°C (284°F).
- In a bowl, toss the kale with olive oil and a pinch of salt until evenly covered.
- Place the kale on two baking pans in a single layer.
- Bake for 15 minutes, then shake the trays and bake for an additional 5-10 minutes until crispy.
- If preferred, sprinkle with additional salt before serving.

Nutritional Information: Calories: 50, Fat: 2.5g, Carbs: 6g, Fiber: 1g, Protein: 2g, Purine Score: Low.

<u>Cucumber and Tomato Salad</u>

- **Servings: four.**
- **Prep time: 10 minutes.**

Ingredients:

- Two medium cucumbers, thinly sliced
- 2 medium tomatoes, sliced into wedges
- 1/4 cup thinly sliced red onion.
- Two teaspoons of olive oil.
- One tablespoon of lemon juice.
- Add salt and pepper to taste.
- Fresh parsley, chopped (optional).

Instructions:

- In a large mixing basin, carefully blend the cucumbers, tomatoes, and red onion.
- Drizzle with olive oil and lemon juice.
- Season with salt and pepper, tossing to mix.
- Garnish with fresh parsley if desired.
- Before serving, let the salad sit for 5 minutes to allow the flavors to mix.

Nutritional Information: Calories: 80, fat: 7g, carbs: 4g, fiber: 1g, protein: 1g, purine score: low.

<u>Roasted Chickpeas.</u>

- **Serves: 8**
- **Prep time: 5 minutes.**
- **Cook for 30-40 minutes.**

Ingredients:

- 2 (15-ounce) cans of chickpeas, rinsed and dried
- Two teaspoons of olive oil.
- 1 ½ teaspoon kosher salt.

Instructions:

- Preheat your oven to 400°F (200°C).
- Dry the chickpeas completely with paper towels.
- Combine the chickpeas, olive oil, and kosher salt.
- Arrange the chickpeas on a baking sheet in a single layer.
- Roast for 20–35 minutes, stirring the pan occasionally, until golden brown and crispy.
- Let cool before serving.

Nutritional Information: Calories: 179, Fat: 6g, Carbs: 27g, Fiber: 5g, Protein: 6g, Purine Score: Low

<u>Apple Slices with Cinnamon.</u>

- **Servings: four.**
- **Prep time: 5 minutes.**
- **Cook time: 25 minutes.**

Ingredients:

- Four medium apples, cored and sliced
- 1 tablespoon unsalted butter melted
- Two teaspoons of brown sugar.
- One teaspoon of ground cinnamon.
- A pinch of nutmeg.

Instructions:

- Preheat the oven to 350°F/175°C.
- Toss apple slices in a large basin with melted butter, brown sugar, cinnamon, and nutmeg until evenly coated.
- Place the apple slices in a single layer on a baking sheet coated with parchment paper.
- Bake for 20-25 minutes, until soft and beginning to caramelise.
- Serve warm.

Nutritional Information: Calories: 115, Fat: 3g, Carbs: 22g, Fiber: 4g, Protein: 0g, Purine Score: Low

Oat Bran Muffins

- **Serves: 12**
- **Prep time: 15 minutes.**
- **Cook time: 15 minutes.**

Ingredients:

- 1 1/2 cups oat bran.
- 1 1/2 cups all-purpose flour.
- 1/2 cup dark brown sugar.
- Two teaspoons of baking powder.
- Two teaspoons of baking soda.
- 1/2 teaspoon salt.
- One cup cooled applesauce.
- Two big eggs.
- 1/4 cup vegetable oil.

Instructions:

- Preheat your oven to 400°F (205°C). Line or grease twelve muffin cups.
- Combine the oat bran, flour, brown sugar, baking powder, baking soda, and salt in a large bowl.
- Combine chilled applesauce, eggs, and oil; stir thoroughly.
- Spoon the batter into the muffin cups.
- Let stand for 10 minutes.
- Bake for approximately 15 minutes, or until golden brown and a toothpick inserted into the center comes out clean.

Nutritional Information: Calories: 182; fat: 6g; carbs: 31g; protein: 5g; purine score: low.

CHAPTER 8: SOUPS AND SALADS

<u>Gout-Safe Vegetable Soup</u>

- **Servings: four.**
- **Prep time: 10 minutes.**
- **Cook for 30 minutes.**

Ingredients:

- One tablespoon of olive oil.
- 1 onion, diced
- 2 garlic cloves, minced
- Two carrots, peeled and chopped
- 2 celery stalks, chopped
- 1 zucchini, diced
- 1 cup green beans (trimmed and chopped into 1-inch pieces)
- Four cups of low-sodium vegetable broth
- 1 can (14.5 oz) chopped tomatoes with no salt added.
- One teaspoon of dried basil
- One teaspoon of dried oregano.
- Add salt and pepper to taste.
- 2 cups spinach, roughly chopped.

Instructions:

- Heat the olive oil in a big pot over medium heat.
- Add the onion and garlic and sauté until transparent.
- Combine carrots, celery, zucchini, and green beans. Cook for five minutes.
- Add in the vegetable broth and diced tomatoes.
- Mix in the basil, oregano, salt, and pepper.

- Bring to a boil, then reduce the heat and simmer for 20 minutes.
- Add the spinach and simmer for another 5 minutes.
- Adjust spice as needed and serve hot.

Nutritional Information: calories: 120, fat: 3g, carbs: 20g, fiber: 5g, protein: 3g, purine score: low.

Carrot and Ginger Soup

- **Servings: four.**
- **Prep time: 10 minutes.**
- **Cook time: 25 minutes.**

Ingredients:

- One tablespoon of olive oil.
- One tiny, chopped onion
- 2 garlic cloves, minced
- 2 teaspoons fresh ginger, grated
- 1 pound of carrots, peeled and chopped
- Four cups of low-sodium vegetable broth
- Add salt and pepper to taste.
- Fresh parsley to garnish.

Instructions:

- Heat the olive oil in a big pot over medium heat.
- Combine onion, garlic, and ginger. Sauté until soft.
- Combine carrots and vegetable broth.
- Season with salt and pepper.

- Bring to a boil, then decrease heat and simmer for 20 minutes, or until carrots are soft.
- Puree the soup using an immersion blender or in batches in a blender until smooth.
- Reheat as needed, sprinkle with parsley, and serve.

Nutrional Information: Calories: 140, fat: 4g, carbs: 24g, fiber: 6g, protein: 2g, purine score: low.

Beetroot and Orange Salad

- **Servings: four.**
- **Prep time: 15 minutes.**

Ingredients:

- 4 medium beets, cooked and sliced
- Two oranges, peeled and segmented
- 1/4 red onion, thinly sliced
- 1/4 cup toasted and chopped walnuts.
- 1/4 cup crumbled feta cheese.
- Two teaspoons of olive oil.
- One tablespoon of balsamic vinegar.
- Add salt and pepper to taste.
- Fresh mint leaves as garnish

Instructions:

- Place the beetroot slices and orange segments on a serving plate.

- Sprinkle with red onion, walnuts, and feta cheese.

• Finish with a drizzle of olive oil and balsamic vinegar.

• Season with salt and pepper.

• Garnish with fresh mint leaves before serving.

Nutritional Information: Calories: 220, fat: 14g, carbs: 20g, fiber: 4g, protein: 6g, purine score: low.

Lentil and Spinach Soup

- **Servings: four.**
- **Prep time: 10 minutes.**
- **Cook for 30 minutes.**

Ingredients:

- One tablespoon of olive oil.
- 1 onion, chopped
- 2 garlic cloves, minced
- 1 cup washed red lentils.
- Four cups of low-sodium vegetable broth
- One teaspoon of ground cumin
- 1/2 teaspoon of ground coriander.
- Add salt and pepper to taste.
- 3 cups fresh spinach, roughly chopped.

Instructions:

- Heat the olive oil in a big pot over medium heat.
- Add the onion and garlic and sauté until tender.
- Combine the lentils, vegetable broth, cumin, and coriander.

- Season with salt and pepper.
- Bring to a boil, then decrease heat and simmer for 20 minutes, or until lentils are cooked.
- Stir in the spinach and simmer for 3 minutes, or until wilted.
- Adjust spice as needed and serve hot.

Nutritional Information: Calories: 230, Fat: 4g, Carbs: 34g, Fiber: 16g, Protein: 14g, Purine Score: Low.

Quinoa Salad with Lemon Dressing

- **Servings: four.**
- **Prep time: 15 minutes.**

Ingredients:

- 2 cups cooked quinoa (cooled)
- One cup cherry tomato, halved
- One cucumber, diced
- 1/4 cup coarsely chopped red onion.
- 1/4 cup chopped parsley.
- 1/4 cup crumbled feta cheese.
- 1/4 cup pitted and sliced kalamata olives.

For lemon dressing:

- Three tablespoons of olive oil.
- 2 teaspoons of lemon juice.
- One teaspoon Dijon mustard.
- One teaspoon of honey.

- Add salt and pepper to taste.

Instructions:

- In a large bowl, combine the quinoa, cherry tomatoes, cucumber, red onion, parsley, feta cheese, and olives.
- In a small mixing bowl, combine the olive oil, lemon juice, mustard, honey, salt, and pepper to make the dressing.
- Toss the salad with the dressing until well combined.
- Serve immediately or refrigerate before serving.

Nutritional Information: Calories: 290, fat: 15g, carbohydrates: 33g, fiber: 5g, protein: 8g, purine score: low

Tomato Soup with Basil

- **Servings: four.**
- **Prep time: 10 minutes.**
- **Cook time: 20 minutes.**

Ingredients:

- 2 pounds of ripe tomatoes, chopped
- 3 garlic cloves, minced
- 1 handful of fresh basil leaves, with extra for garnish.
- 1 tablespoon tomato purée.
- 2 tablespoons olive oil.
- Four cups of low-sodium vegetable broth
- Add salt and freshly ground black pepper to taste.
- 1-2 tablespoons sugar (to taste)

- One-half cup light cream

Instructions:

- Warm the olive oil in a big pot over medium heat.
- Cook the chopped tomatoes for 5 minutes, or until they begin to soften.
- Add the garlic, basil, and tomato purée and simmer for another 2 minutes.
- Pour in the veggie broth and bring to a boil before simmering for 15 minutes.
- Using an immersion blender or a normal blender, mix the soup until it is smooth.
- Return the soup to the pot, seasoning with salt, pepper, and sugar.
- Stir in the cream and heat through without boiling.
- Garnish with fresh basil leaves.

Nutritional Information: Calories: 200, fat: 14g, carbs: 17g, fiber: 3g, protein: 3g, purine score: low.

Mixed Greens and Apple Cider Vinaigrette

- **Servings: four.**
- **Prep time: 10 minutes.**

Ingredients:

- Eight cups of mixed greens
- One apple, thinly sliced
- 1/4 cup toasted pecans.

For the vinaigrette:

- 1 clove garlic, minced
- 2 teaspoons Dijon mustard.

- 1 tablespoon honey.
- 3–4 tablespoons apple cider vinegar
- One-third cup olive oil
- Add salt and pepper to taste.

Instructions:

- In a large mixing bowl, add mixed greens, apple slices, and toasted pecans.
- In a small bowl, combine garlic, mustard, honey, vinegar, and olive oil to make the vinaigrette dressing. Season with salt and pepper.
- Drizzle the vinaigrette over the salad right before serving and toss to coat evenly.

Nutritional Information: Calories: 250, fat: 21g, carbohydrates: 18g, fiber: 3g, protein: 2g, purine score: low.

Cabbage Slaw with Apples

- **Servings: six.**
- **Prep time: 15 minutes.**

Ingredients:

- 1 small head cabbage, finely chopped
- One Granny Smith apple, sliced into matchsticks.
- 1/2 cup of apple cider vinegar.
- 1/2 cup of white sugar.
- 3 tablespoons olive oil.
- One tablespoon Dijon mustard
- 1/4 teaspoon of red pepper flakes

Instructions:

- Combine cabbage and apples in a big basin.
- In a saucepan, combine vinegar, sugar, olive oil, mustard, and red pepper flakes; heat to a simmer.
- Toss the cabbage mixture with the heated dressing until coated.
- Refrigerate for at least one hour before serving.

Nutritional Information: Calories: 141, Fat: 8g, Carbs: 17g, Protein: 1g, Purine Score: Low.

<u>Orange and Walnut Salad</u>

- **Servings: four.**
- **Prep time: 15 minutes.**

Ingredients:

- 10 ounces mixed salad greens.
- Two large navel oranges, peeled and sectioned
- 1/2 cup of sliced red onion.
- 3/4 cup roasted walnut halves.
- 1/4 cup of crumbled Gorgonzola

For Dressing:

- One-quarter cup olive oil
- 2 tablespoons balsamic vinegar.
- 2 teaspoons Dijon mustard.
- 1/4 teaspoon of dried oregano.
- Add salt and pepper to taste.

Instructions:

- In a large salad bowl, mix together the lettuce, oranges, red onion, and toasted walnuts.
- In a container, combine olive oil, vinegar, mustard, oregano, salt, and pepper. Shake well.
- Drizzle the dressing over the salad, then mix.
- Sprinkle with Gorgonzola cheese and serve.

Nutritional Information: calories: 368, fat: 30g, carbs: 23g, protein: 5g, purine score: low.

CHAPTER 9: DRINKS AND SMOOTHIES.

Pineapple and Banana Smoothie

- **Servings: two.**
- **Prep time: 5 minutes.**

Ingredients:

- One cup of frozen pineapple pieces.
- 1 ripe banana (ideally frozen)
- One cup unsweetened almond milk.
- Optional: 1 tablespoon honey, to taste.

Instructions:

- Combine the pineapple, banana, and almond milk in a blender.
- Blend on high until smooth and creamy.
- Taste and add honey if you prefer a sweeter smoothie.
- Serve immediately.

Nutritional Information: Calories: 180, fat: 1.5g, carbohydrates: 44g, fiber: 5g, protein: 2g, purine score: low.

<u>Lemon & Ginger Tea</u>

- **Servings: two.**
- **Prep time: 5 minutes.**
- **Cook for 5 minutes.**

Ingredients:

- One lemon.
- Thinly slice 2 inches of fresh ginger.
- Two cups of boiling water.
- Honey to taste is optional.

Instructions:

- Squeeze the lemon juice into a heatproof teapot or pitcher.
- Add the sliced ginger and lemon juice to the saucepan.
- Pour in the boiling water and steep for approximately 5 minutes.
- Strain the tea into mugs and add honey if desired.

Nutritional Information: Calories: 19; fat: 0.1g; carbs: 6g; fiber: 0.5g; protein: 0.2g; purine score: low.

Cherry Smoothie with Almond Milk.

- **Servings: two.**
- **Prep time: 5 minutes.**

Ingredients:

- One cup frozen cherry.
- One ripe banana.
- One cup unsweetened almond milk.
- Optional: 1 tablespoon almond butter.

Instructions:

- Mix the cherries, banana, and almond milk in a blender.
- Blend until smooth.
- If using almond butter, add it and continue to combine.
- Serve immediately.

Nutritional Information: Calories: 150, Fat: 3g, Carbs: 28g, Fiber: 4g, Protein: 2g, Purine Score: Low.

<u>**Watermelon with Mint Juice**</u>

- **Servings: four.**
- **Prep time: 10 minutes.**

Ingredients:

- 4 cups of cubed seedless watermelon, cold
- 1/4 cup of fresh mint leaves.
- One lime, juiced

Instructions:

- Combine watermelon cubes, mint leaves, and lime juice in a blender.
- Blend until smooth.
- Pass through a fine mesh sieve into a pitcher.
- Pour over ice and garnish with extra mint leaves if preferred.

Nutritional Information: Calories: 60, fat: 0.5g, carbs: 15g, fiber: 1g, protein: 1g, purine score: low.

Cucumber-Lime Infused Water

- **Servings: four.**
- **Prep time: 5 minutes.**

Ingredients:

- One medium cucumber, thinly sliced
- One lime, thinly sliced
- Eight cups of water.
- Ice cubes.

Instructions:

- In a large pitcher, mix together the cucumber and lime slices.
- Fill the pitcher with water and add some ice cubes.
- Refrigerate for at least one hour to let the flavors to mingle.
- Serve cold.

<u>**Peach and Yogurt Smoothie**</u>

- **Servings: two.**
- **Prep time: 5 minutes.**

Ingredients:

- 3 cups sliced peaches, fresh or frozen.
- One cup of Greek yogurt.
- 1 cup almond milk, frozen in an ice cube tray.
- Two teaspoons of honey (optional).

Instructions:

- Blend the peaches, Greek yogurt, and almond milk until smooth.
- If you want it sweeter, add honey.
- Serve immediately and enjoy!

Nutritional Information: Calories: 309, Fat: 7g, Carbs: 49g, Protein: 11g, Purine Score: Low.

Herbal Tea with Honey.

- **Servings: two.**
- **Prep time: 5 minutes.**
- **Cook time: 15 minutes.**

Ingredients:

- 1 tablespoon of your favorite dry herbs, such as chamomile, mint, or ginger.
- Two cups of boiling water.
- Honey to taste.

Instructions:

- Transfer the dry herbs to a teapot or heatproof pitcher.
- Pour the boiling water over the herbs and steep for approximately 15 minutes.
- Strain the tea into mugs and sweeten with honey as desired.

Nutritional Information: Calories: 64 (with 1 tablespoon honey), Fat: 0g, Carbs: 17g, Fiber: 0g, Protein: 0g, Purine Score: Low.

<u>Coconut Water with A Splash of Lime</u>

- **Serves: 1**
- **Prep time: 2 minutes.**

Ingredients:

- One cup of coconut water.
- Juice from 1/2 lime.
- Ice cubes.

Instructions:

- Fill a glass with ice cubes.
- Pour coconut water over the ice.
- Squeeze half a lime into the glass.
- Stir thoroughly and serve cold.

Nutritional Information: Calories: 46, fat: 0g, carbs: 9g, fiber: 2.6g, protein: 1.7g, purine score: low.

<u>**Berry and Spinach Smoothie**</u>

- **Servings: two.**
- **Prep time: 5 minutes.**

Ingredients:

- 1 cup mixed berries (strawberries, raspberries, blueberries)
- One ripe banana.
- One cup baby spinach.
- One spoonful of chia seeds.
- One cup of almond milk.

Instructions:

- Combine all ingredients in a blender.
- Blend on high until smooth and creamy.
- Serve immediately.

Nutritional Information: Calories: 145, Fat: 4g, Carbs: 27g, Fiber: 7g, Protein: 3g, Purine Score: Low

<u>**Baked Apples with Cinnamon.**</u>

- **Servings: four.**
- **Prep time: 10 minutes.**
- **Cook for 30 minutes.**

Ingredients:

- Four big, cored apples
- 2 teaspoons cinnamon.
- 4 teaspoons honey.
- One-quarter cup water

Instructions:

- Preheat the oven to 350°F/175°C.
- Place the cored apples into a baking dish.
- Fill the center of each apple with 1/2 teaspoon cinnamon and 1 teaspoon honey.
- Pour water into the bottom of the dish.
- Bake the apples for 30 minutes, or until soft and tender.
- Serve warm.

Nutritional Information: Calories: 95, fat: 0.3g, carbs: 25g, fiber: 4.4g, protein: 0.5g, purine score: low.

<u>**Yogurt Parfait with Fresh Berries.**</u>

- **Servings: two.**
- **Prep time: 5 minutes.**

Ingredients:

- Two cups of Greek yogurt.
- One cup of fresh berries (strawberries, blueberries, raspberries).
- 1/4 cup granola.
- Honey for drizzling (optional)

Instructions:

- In serving glasses, add 1/2 cup yogurt, then a layer of mixed berries.
- Add a tablespoon of granola to the berries.
- Repeat the layers until the glasses are full.
- Drizzle with honey if desired.
- Serve immediately or chill until ready to use.

Nutritional Information: Calories: 150, fat: 2g, carbs: 20g, fiber: 2g, protein: 10g, purine score: low.

Chia Seed Pudding with Coconut Milk

- **Servings: four.**
- **Prep time is 5 minutes (plus soaking time).**

Ingredients:

- 1/4 cup of chia seeds.
- One cup of coconut milk.
- One tablespoon of honey or maple syrup.
- Fresh fruit as a topping

Instructions:

- In a bowl, combine the chia seeds and coconut milk.
- Stir in the honey or maple syrup.
- Cover and refrigerate for at least 2 hours, or overnight, until the mixture thickens to a pudding consistency.
- Garnish with fresh fruit before serving.

Nutritional Information: Calories: 130, Fat: 8g, Carbs: 12g, Fiber: 5g, Protein: 3g, Purine Score: Low.

Almond and Cherry Clafoutis.

- **Servings: six.**
- **Prep time: 15 minutes.**
- **Cook time: 35 minutes.**

Ingredients:

- One-half cup almond flour
- One-quarter cup sugar
- 3 eggs
- One cup of almond milk.
- 1 teaspoon of almond extract.
- Two cups of pitted cherries

Instructions:

- Preheat the oven to 350°F/175°C.
- In a mixing bowl, combine almond flour, sugar, eggs, almond milk, and almond extract. Whisk until smooth.
- Transfer the batter to a prepared baking tray.
- Distribute the pitted cherries equally on top.
- Bake for 35 minutes, or until firm and lightly brown.
- Serve warm.

Nutritional Information: Calories: 180, fat: 10g, carbohydrates: 18g, fiber: 3g, protein: 6g, purine score: low.

<u>Fruit Sorbet</u>

- **Servings: four.**
- **Preparation time: 10 minutes (including freezing time)**

Ingredients:

- 4 cups of fresh fruit (berries, mango, or peach)
- 1/2 cup sugar (or honey)
- 2 tablespoons lemon juice.

Instructions:

- Using a blender, puree the fruit until smooth.
- Mix in the sugar or honey and lemon juice.
- Transfer the mixture to a shallow dish and freeze until hard, about 4 hours.
- Allow the sorbet to soften briefly at room temperature before serving.
- Serve sorbet in bowls or cones.

Nutritional Information: Calories: 160, fat: 0g, carbohydrates: 40g, fiber: 3g, protein: 1g, purine score: low

Poached Pears in Spiced Tea

- **Servings: four.**
- **Prep time: 10 minutes.**
- **Cook time: 20 minutes.**

Ingredients:

- Four ripe, peeled pears
- Four cups of water.
- Four spicy tea bags (chai or equivalent).
- One cinnamon stick.
- Two-star anise.
- One-quarter cup honey

Instructions:

- In a large pot, heat the water to a boil, then add the tea bags, cinnamon stick, and star anise.
- Reduce the heat and simmer for 5 minutes to infuse the spices.
- Put the pears and honey into the pot.
- Simmer gently for 15-20 minutes, or until the pears are softened.
- Remove the pears and allow them to cool.
- Drizzle the pears with the spiced tea syrup.

Nutritional Information: Calories: 180, fat: 0g, carbs: 47g, fiber: 6g, protein: 0.5g, purine score: low.

<u>Carrot Oatmeal Muffins</u>

- **Serves: 12**
- **Prep time: 15 minutes.**
- **Cook time: 20 minutes.**

Ingredients:

- One cup whole wheat flour.
- One cup rolled oats.
- One-half cup brown sugar
- 2 teaspoons baking powder.
- 1/2 teaspoon baking soda.
- 1/4 teaspoon salt.
- One teaspoon of cinnamon.
- 1/2 teaspoon nutmeg.
- One cup shredded carrot.
- 3/4 cup unsweetened applesauce.
- One-half cup vegetable oil
- 2 eggs
- 1 teaspoon of vanilla extract.

Instructions:

- Preheat the oven to 350°F/175°C and line a muffin tray with paper liners.
- In a large mixing bowl, combine the flour, oats, brown sugar, baking powder, soda, salt, cinnamon, and nutmeg.
- Stir in the grated carrots.
- In a separate dish, whisk together the applesauce, oil, eggs, and vanilla.
- Mix the wet and dry ingredients until barely combined.
- Fill each muffin cup 3/4 full and bake for 20 minutes, or until a toothpick comes out clean.
- Allow the muffins to cool before serving.

Nutritional Information: Calories: 190, Fat: 10g, Carbs: 23g, Fiber: 3g, Protein: 3g, Purine Score: Low

<u>**Berry Compote with Whipped Cream**</u>

- **Servings: four.**
- **Prep time: 5 minutes.**
- **Cooking Time: 10 minutes.**

Ingredients:

- Two cups mixed berries (strawberries, blueberries, raspberries)
- One-quarter cup sugar
- One tablespoon of lemon juice.
- One cup heavy cream.
- One tablespoon of powdered sugar.

Instructions:

- In a saucepan, mix the berries, sugar, and lemon juice.
- Cook for about 10 minutes over medium heat, or until the berries have broken down and the sauce has thickened.
- In a mixing basin, combine the heavy cream and powdered sugar. Whisk until soft peaks form.
- Top the warm berry compote with a dollop of whipped cream.

Nutritional information: calories: 315, fat: 22g, carbs: 29g, fiber: 3g, protein: 2g, purine score: low.

<u>Pineapple and Mango Salad</u>

- **Servings: four.**
- **Prep time: 15 minutes.**

Ingredients:

- One cup diced pineapple.
- One cup chopped mango.
- 1/4 cup of thinly sliced red onion.
- 1/4 cup of chopped cilantro.
- Juice from 1 lime
- Add salt and pepper to taste.

Instructions:

- In a bowl, combine the pineapple, mango, red onion, and cilantro.
- Drizzle lime juice over the mixture and season with salt and pepper.
- Combine everything and refrigerate in the refrigerator for at least 30 minutes before serving.

Nutritional Information: Calories: 95, fat: 0.5g, carbs: 24g, fiber: 3g, protein: 1g, purine score: low.

CHAPTER 11: BONUS SECTION

The 28-Day Gout Diet Plan

Week 1:

Day 1:

- Breakfast: oatmeal with sliced peaches and almond butter.
- Lunch: Mixed salad with cottage cheese and chives.
- Dinner: Grilled salmon with a side of asparagus

Day 2:

- Breakfast: Scrambled eggs, spinach, and mushrooms.
- Lunch: Egg Salad Sandwich with Whole Wheat Bread
- Dinner: Chicken and broccoli casserole with cherries and almonds

Day 3:

- Breakfast: Whole wheat toast with avocado spread.
- Lunch: Lentil soup with carrots and celery.
- Dinner: Vegetable Stir-Fry with Tofu.

Day 4:

- Breakfast: cottage cheese with pineapple chunks.
- Lunch: Quinoa and black bean salad.
- Dinner: Baked trout with herb seasoning.

Day 5:

- Breakfast: Banana and cherry smoothie.
- Lunch: Veggie wrap with hummus and cucumber.
- Dinner: Roasted turkey breast with green beans.

Day 6:

- Breakfast: Buckwheat pancakes with apple compote.
- Lunch: baked cod with lemon and dill.
- Dinner: Shrimp and vegetable kabobs.

Day 7:

- Breakfast: Quinoa porridge with almonds and blueberries.
- Lunch: stuffed bell peppers with brown rice and vegetables.
- Dinner: Lentil and vegetable curry.

Week 2:

Day 8:

- Breakfast: Baked sweet potatoes with cinnamon and nutmeg.
- Lunch: Mixed salad with cottage cheese and chives.
- Dinner: Grilled salmon with a side of asparagus

Day 9:

- Breakfast: Chia Seed Pudding and Fresh Fruit.
- Lunch: Egg Salad Sandwich with Whole Wheat Bread
- Dinner: chicken and broccoli casserole with cherries and almonds.

Day 10:

- Breakfast: oatmeal with sliced peaches and almond butter.
- Lunch: Lentil soup with carrots and celery.
- Dinner: Vegetable Stir-Fry with Tofu.

Day 11:

- Breakfast: Scrambled eggs, spinach, and mushrooms.
- Lunch: Quinoa and black bean salad.
- Dinner: Baked trout with herb seasoning.

Day 12:

- Breakfast: Whole wheat toast with avocado spread.
- Lunch: Veggie wrap with hummus and cucumber.
- Dinner: Roasted turkey breast with green beans.

Day 13:

- Breakfast: cottage cheese with pineapple chunks.
- Lunch: baked cod with lemon and dill.
- Dinner: Shrimp and vegetable kabobs.

Day 14:

- Breakfast: Banana and cherry smoothie.
- Lunch is stuffed bell peppers with brown rice and vegetables.
- Dinner: Lentil and vegetable curry.

Week 3:

Day 15:

- Breakfast: Chia Seed Pudding and Fresh Fruit.
- Lunch: Mixed salad with cottage cheese and chives.
- Dinner: Grilled salmon with a side of asparagus

Day 16:

- Breakfast: Buckwheat pancakes with apple compote.
- Lunch: Egg Salad Sandwich with Whole Wheat Bread
- Dinner: chicken and broccoli casserole with cherries and almonds.

Day 17:

- Breakfast: Quinoa porridge with almonds and blueberries.
- Lunch: Lentil soup with carrots and celery.
- Dinner: Vegetable Stir-Fry with Tofu.

Day 18:

- Breakfast: Baked sweet potatoes with cinnamon and nutmeg.
- Lunch: Quinoa and black bean salad.
- Dinner: Baked trout with herb seasoning.

Day 19:

- Breakfast: oatmeal with sliced peaches and almond butter.
- Lunch: Veggie wrap with hummus and cucumber.
- Dinner: Roasted turkey breast with green beans.

Day 20:

- Breakfast: Scrambled eggs, spinach, and mushrooms.
- Lunch: baked cod with lemon and dill.
- Dinner: Shrimp and vegetable kabobs.

Day 21:

- Breakfast: Whole wheat toast with avocado spread.
- Lunch: stuffed bell peppers with brown rice and vegetables.
- Dinner: Lentil and vegetable curry.

Week 4:

Day 22:

- Breakfast: cottage cheese with pineapple chunks.
- Lunch: Mixed salad with cottage cheese and chives.
- Dinner: Grilled salmon with a side of asparagus

Day 23:

- Breakfast: Banana and cherry smoothie.
- Lunch: Egg Salad Sandwich with Whole Wheat Bread
- Dinner: chicken and broccoli casserole with cherries and almonds.

Day 24:

- Breakfast: Buckwheat pancakes with apple compote.
- Lunch: Lentil soup with carrots and celery.
- Dinner: Vegetable Stir-Fry with Tofu.

Day 25:

- Breakfast: Quinoa porridge with almonds and blueberries.
- Lunch: Quinoa and black bean salad.
- Dinner: Baked trout with herb seasoning.

Day 26:

- Breakfast: Baked sweet potatoes with cinnamon and nutmeg.
- Lunch: Veggie wrap with hummus and cucumber.
- Dinner: Roasted turkey breast with green beans.

Day 27:

- Breakfast: Chia Seed Pudding and Fresh Fruit.
- Lunch: baked cod with lemon and dill.
- Dinner: Shrimp and vegetable kabobs.

Day 28:

- Breakfast: oatmeal with sliced peaches and almond butter.
- Lunch: stuffed bell peppers with brown rice and vegetables.
- Dinner: Lentil and vegetable curry.

<u>Living With Gout</u>

Living with gout entails more than just monitoring your diet; it necessitates a comprehensive approach to lifestyle that includes exercise, stress management, and other healthy activities.

- **Regular physical exercise** is good for your overall health and can help you manage your gout by keeping you at a healthy weight and lowering your risk of chronic diseases that can aggravate your symptoms. Aim to complete at least 150 minutes of moderate-intensity aerobic activity per week, such as brisk walking or swimming. Avoid high-impact exercises that can cause joint stress during a gout flare-up.
- **Stress Management**: Because stress can lead to gout episodes, it is critical to discover appropriate stress management techniques. Deep breathing, meditation, yoga, and tai chi are all effective techniques. Additionally, engaging in hobbies and activities that you enjoy might help to alleviate stress.
- **Adequate Rest and Sleep**: Getting enough sleep is essential for good health and can assist with gout. Poor sleep can raise the body's stress and inflammatory levels, potentially leading to more frequent gout attacks. Aim for 7-9 hours of quality sleep per night.
- **Maintain a Healthy Weight**: Being overweight increases the likelihood of gout episodes. Gradual weight loss with a well-balanced diet and regular exercise will help lower uric acid levels and prevent gout attacks.
- **Consider Herbal and Dietary Supplements**: Certain herbal and dietary supplements may help alleviate gout symptoms. However, always ask your doctor before starting any new supplement, since some may interfere with medications or have negative effects.

- **Alternative Treatments and Natural Remedies**: Trying alternative treatments like acupuncture or massage therapy may help relieve gout symptoms. Natural therapies, such as ingesting cherries or cherry extract, have been linked to less gout attacks, though additional research is needed.

- **Regular Medical Checkups**: Regular visits to your healthcare provider are essential for monitoring your condition and making any required changes to your treatment plan.

By making these lifestyle adjustments, you can help your gout diet and live a healthy life while controlling your illness. Remember that these are broad ideas, and it is always preferable to contact with a healthcare professional for guidance customized to your specific need.

FAQs

- **What is gout, and what causes it?** Gout is a type of inflammatory arthritis that causes sudden and intense pain, redness, and swelling in the joints, usually affecting the big toe. Elevated amounts of uric acid in the blood can lead to the formation of crystals in the joints.

- **How does the diet impact gout?** Diet is important in managing gout because certain meals can raise uric acid levels in the blood. Foods heavy in purines, such as red meat and shellfish, should be limited. A diet rich in fruits, vegetables, whole grains, and low-fat dairy products can help regulate uric acid levels.

- **Are there any things I should avoid to prevent gout flare-ups?** Yes, it is advisable to avoid or limit meals high in purines, such as organ meats, some seafood, and alcoholic beverages, particularly beer. Instead, prioritize low-purine foods such as fruits, vegetables, and whole grains.

- **Can decreasing weight assist with gout treatment**? Yes, keeping a healthy weight can help limit the number of gout attacks. Gradual weight loss with a balanced diet and regular exercise is encouraged, but crash diets should be avoided because they can increase uric acid levels.

- **Is exercise safe for gout sufferers**? Exercise is generally safe and useful for gout sufferers. It can aid in maintaining a healthy weight and lowering the risk of chronic diseases that can exacerbate gout symptoms. However, during a gout attack, it's better not to put pressure on the affected joints.

- **If I have gout, how much water should I drink**? Staying hydrated is crucial for eliminating uric acid from the body. Drink at least 8 cups of fluids every day, primarily water, unless directed otherwise by your healthcare provider.

- **Can I consume wine if I have gout**? Alcohol use, especially beer, can raise uric acid levels and cause gout attacks. It's better to minimize or avoid alcohol, and if you do decide to drink, choose wine in moderation.

- **Are there any natural treatments for gout**? Some natural therapies, such as ingesting cherries or cherry extract, have been linked to less gout attacks. However, additional study is needed, and you should talk with your healthcare professional before trying any new treatments.

- **Should I use gout medications**? Medication can be an important aspect of gout management, particularly during flare-ups or to regulate uric acid levels over time. Always talk about drug options with your healthcare provider.

CONCLUSION

As we conclude our culinary journey, I hope that "The Gout Diet Cookbook" has offered you with not just a selection of tasty recipes, but also a new perspective on gout management through diet and lifestyle. The decisions we make at the dinner table frequently pave the way to wellbeing, and this book has been designed to make that journey as simple and enjoyable as possible.

Your health and contentment are really important, and I feel that the meals you've discovered here will not only delight your taste buds but also contribute to your overall well-being. If you've found consolation in these dishes and added comfort to your table, I'd appreciate it if you could share your thoughts.

Positive feedback and honest reviews are really valuable. They assist others who are facing similar issues in finding trust in these pages, and, more significantly, they enable for the ongoing enhancement of this resource. If you have a moment, please consider leaving a review where you purchased the book or on any platform of your choice. Your views and experiences can make a huge impact in someone else's gout treatment.

Thank you for making this cookbook a part of your kitchen and lifestyle. May your meals be savory, your health strong, and your days filled with the delight of sharing wonderful food with loved ones.

I wish you a life of health and happiness.